NORDIC WALKING THERAPY

Revitalize Your Body And Mind, A Comprehensive Guide To Harnessing Nature's Cure For Fitness, Stress Relief, And Total Well-Being

DR. WANDA MENDENHALL

DISCLAIMER

This book is the result of the author's own expertise, insight, and experience in the area of treatment. The author has no affiliation with any particular firm, business, or person mentioned in this article. The content in this book is based exclusively on the author's knowledge and should not be construed as professional advice or a replacement for professional treatment or counseling.

Readers are recommended to seek professional counsel or guidance based on their unique circumstances or requirements. The author and publisher are not liable for any actions done in reliance on the information included in this book. Every person's circumstance is unique, so what works for one person may not work for another.

This book attempts to provide insights and knowledge for both education and personal growth.

The author does not recommend any certain therapy strategy or practice over another. Readers should exercise caution and check with trained specialists before using any knowledge or strategies discussed in this book.

By reading this book, the reader understands and accepts that the author and publisher are not accountable for any direct or indirect repercussions, damages, or losses that occur from the use or misuse of the material included herein.

Table of Contents

CHAPTER ONE

Introduction

Understanding Nordic Walking Therapy

Nordic Walking Therapy is a novel and revolutionary method for physical and emotional well-being that integrates Nordic walking principles with treatments. Nordic walking, which began as a summer training technique for cross-country skiers in Finland in the 1. 9. . 3. 0s, has now grown into a popular kind of fitness exercise worldwide. What distinguishes Nordic Walking Therapy is its purposeful use of therapeutic aspects to improve overall wellness.

Nordic walking has its origins in Finland, where cross-country skiers employed it to maintain their fitness levels during the off-season. Because the action engages the upper, lower, and core muscles, it has been recognized as a good full-body workout. Nordic walking evolved from a training strategy for athletes to a leisure and fitness activity for individuals of all ages and fitness levels throughout time.

Nordic walking's therapeutic adaption arose as a natural step, recognizing its comprehensive advantages. Walking with poles not only improves cardiovascular fitness but also gives stability and support, making it accessible to people of all physical abilities. Nordic Walking Therapy evolved to meet particular therapeutic requirements such as rehabilitation, stress reduction, and mental health enhancement as it gained popularity.

Benefits And Significance In Physical And Mental Well-Being

Nordic Walking Therapy has several physical and emotional advantages, making it a flexible intervention in the domain of holistic health.

Physical Advantages:

1. *.Cardiovascular Fitness:* Nordic walking's rhythmic arm and leg motions activate

key muscle groups, increasing cardiovascular health and endurance.

2. *.Muscle Engagement:* Unlike typical walking, Nordic walking uses poles to activate muscles in the arms, shoulders, and core, providing a more thorough exercise.

3. .The use of poles decreases the stress on joints, making it a low-impact exercise suited for those with arthritis or joint problems.

4. *.Caloric Expenditure:* When compared to conventional walking, Nordic walking has been demonstrated to boost caloric expenditure, which aids with weight control and fitness objectives.

Mental Health Advantages:

1.   *.tension Reduction:* Nordic walking's rhythmic nature, along with the connection to nature, has a relaxing impact, lowering tension and fostering relaxation.

2. *.Improved Mood:* Regular Nordic Walking Therapy participation has been linked to the production of endorphins, which contribute to a happy mood and a feeling of well-being.

3.   .Group Nordic walking sessions promote social well-being and develop a sense of community, minimizing feelings of loneliness.

4.   *.Cognitive Benefits:* The coordination necessary for Nordic walking may improve cognitive performance by improving attention and executive functioning.

Finally, Nordic Walking Therapy is a synthesis of physical exercise and therapeutic ideas that provide a comprehensive approach to health and well-being. This introductory chapter serves as a foundation for a more in-depth examination of the history, development, and many advantages of this novel therapeutic technique.

CHAPTER TWO

The Fundamentals Of Nordic Walking

Nordic Walking Therapy is a kind of exercise that combines the advantages of walking with the use of specially built poles. We will go into the fundamentals of Nordic Walking in this chapter, concentrating on basic skills, equipment, appropriate posture, body mechanics, and selecting the best poles for individual requirements.

Basic Techniques And Equipment

1. . Holding the Poles:
Gripping the Nordic walking poles correctly is critical for efficient technique. Gripping the handles with a strong yet

relaxed grasp aids in the effective transmission of power during each stride. The pole straps should be adjusted to offer support and allow for a natural arm swing.

2. . Stride and arm swing:

Nordic Walking is distinguished by a characteristic arm swing that utilizes the upper body muscles. The coordination of the arm swing and stride improves the total cardiovascular and muscular advantages. The poles are placed behind the walker's torso, and when he or she steps forward with one foot, the opposing arm swings forward.

3. . Pole Planting Method:

The poles are placed diagonally behind the torso, allowing for a natural and efficient energy transmission. The proper angle of pole planting provides stability and aids in propelling the walker ahead. Novice walkers may need considerable work to learn arm and leg coordination.

4. . Terrain for Walking:

Nordic Walking may be done on a variety of terrains, such as flat ground, hills, and rough pathways. Adjusting the approach according to the terrain gives a full-body exercise and optimizes muscle activation.

5. . Breathing Method:

Proper breathing is an important part of Nordic Walking. Coordination of the breath with the arm swing and stride improves oxygen intake and energy production. Deep, regular breathing improves endurance and promotes calm during physical exercise.

6. . Overview of the Equipment:

Nordic walking poles are particularly intended for this sport. They are longer than standard walking poles and include ergonomic grips and straps. The poles may also have shock-absorbing mechanisms to lessen joint impact. It is important to choose poles that are appropriate for one's height and fitness level.

1. . Alignment of the Body:

Proper body alignment is essential for injury prevention and peak performance. Nordic walkers should stand tall, with a straight back, relaxed shoulders, and engaged core muscles. The poles help to maintain balance and stability.

2. . Primary Engagement:

Each step gains stability and strength by using the core muscles. Nordic Walking's circular upper-body motions stimulate the core, resulting in a full-body exercise and improved posture.

3. . Foot Positioning:

Paying attention to foot positioning aids in weight distribution and lowers joint tension. Nordic walkers should land on their heels and roll their feet through to their toes to provide a natural and comfortable stride.

Choosing The Right Poles For Your Needs

1. . Pole Dimensions:

Nordic walking pole length is critical for optimal technique. Poles should be chosen depending on a person's height, with a rough rule of thumb stating that poles should be 70-8. 0% of a person's height.

2. . Weight and material:

Nordic walking poles are often composed of lightweight materials like aluminum or carbon fiber. The weight of the poles is affected by the material used, and walkers should choose a weight that is comfortable for prolonged usage.

3. . Grip and Strap Specifications:

Comfort and control are enhanced with ergonomic grips and adjustable straps. Grips should be comfortable to wear, and adjustable straps should be large enough to give a secure but flexible connection between the hands and poles.

4. . Absorption of Shock:
Some Nordic walking poles include shock absorption properties. This might be advantageous for those who have joint issues or desire a milder sensation during each pole plant.

Finally, learning the principles of Nordic Walking, such as basic methods, good posture, body mechanics, and equipment selection, is critical for optimizing the therapeutic effects of this exercise. Nordic Walking is an adaptable and fun method of physical exercise that may be used for fitness, rehabilitation, or general well-being.

CHAPTER THREE

Physiological Impact Of Nordic Walking

Nordic Walking Therapy is a comprehensive method of exercise that combines the advantages of walking with the use of specially built poles. The physiological effect of Nordic Walking will be examined in this chapter, with an emphasis on three main aspects: Cardiovascular Benefits, Muscular Engagement and Strength Building, and effect on Joint Health and Flexibility.

Cardiovascular Benefits

1. **.Aerobic Exercise:** Nordic Walking engages more muscle areas than typical walking since it uses both the upper and

lower body. This increased muscular engagement raises the heart rate and improves cardiovascular health. Nordic Walking's rhythmic and fluid action promotes aerobic exercise, boosting the efficiency of oxygen use, and promoting cardiovascular health.

2.   .Nordic Walking has been found in studies to boost caloric expenditure when compared to conventional walking. Using poles increases resistance, which requires more energy and results in a bigger calorie burn. As a result, Nordic Walking is a beneficial exercise for weight loss and general cardiovascular fitness.

3.   .**Improved Blood Circulation:** Nordic Walking's mix of arm and leg motions improves blood circulation throughout the body. This enhanced circulation benefits the cardiovascular system by improving oxygen supply to muscles and organs. Improved blood flow may help to reduce the risk of cardiovascular disease.

Muscular Engagement And Strength Building

1.   .**Total Body Workout:** Nordic Walking works a variety of muscles in the arms, shoulders, core, and lower body. This full total-body exercise is provided by this holistic method. The poles' continual push and pull action activates muscles that may be neglected in conventional walking,

resulting in increased physical strength and endurance.

2.   .Core Stability is required for the process of moving oneself forward with the poles. This regular activation of the core muscles not only improves posture but also develops the abdominal and back muscles. A solid core is necessary for overall stability and balance.

3.   .**Upper Body Strength:** Unlike regular walking, which focuses on the lower body, Nordic Walking focuses on the upper body. This strengthens the arms, shoulders, and chest muscles. Individuals may see increased upper body strength and tone with time.

1.   .Nordic Walking is a low-impact workout that is kinder on the joints than high-impact activities such as jogging. The use of poles relieves strain on the knees, hips, and lower back, making it an ideal solution for those who have joint problems or arthritis.

2.   **.Improved Joint Flexibility:** The full-body motions included in Nordic Walking help to enhance joint flexibility. Regular practice aids in the maintenance and improvement of range of motion in the shoulders, elbows, hips, and knees. This may be especially good for elderly people or those healing from joint issues.

3. .**Balanced Muscular Development:** Nordic Walking promotes a balanced effort allocation between the upper and lower bodies. By minimizing muscle imbalances that might lead to joint disorders, this balance helps general joint health. Nordic Walking's regulated and symmetrical motions encourage joint-friendly exercise.

Finally, Nordic Walking Therapy provides a holistic approach to enhancing physiological well-being. It is a great therapeutic tool for persons seeking a comprehensive and effective type of physical exercise because of the cardiovascular advantages, muscle engagement, and favorable influence on joint health and flexibility.

CHAPTER FOUR

Mental And Emotional Well-Being

Mental and emotional well-being is an important element of overall health, and Nordic Walking's function in encouraging a pleasant frame of mind is becoming more recognized. This chapter digs into the link between Nordic Walking treatment and mental and emotional well-being, concentrating on stress reduction, the relationship between exercise and mental health, and the cognitive advantages of participating in outdoor activities.

Stress is a natural component of contemporary life, and its negative impacts on mental and emotional health are well-documented. Nordic Walking is an excellent stress management therapy due to its unique blend of physical exercise and absorption in nature.

Physical Activity and Stress Chemicals: Physical activity, such as Nordic Walking, causes the release of endorphins, or "feel-good" chemicals. These hormones function as natural stress relievers, reducing tension and improving mood. Furthermore, the rhythmic, repeated nature of Nordic

Walking generates a contemplative state, which reduces stress levels even further.

Nature Connection: Nordic Walking puts people outside, giving them the chance to connect with nature. The tranquil setting, fresh air, and natural surroundings all add to a feeling of serenity and relaxation, serving as a counterweight to the hurry and bustle of everyday life.

Social component: The social component of Nordic Walking aids with stress relief. Participating in this activity in a group environment promotes a supportive community, allowing people to share their experiences and make new relationships. Social contacts have been shown to improve mental health and contribute to stress reduction.

Connection Between Exercise And Mental Health

Neurobiological Mechanisms: Exercise, particularly Nordic Walking, has a significant impact on the neurobiological functioning of the brain. Regular physical exercise boosts the production of neurotransmitters related to mood control and emotional well-being, such as serotonin and dopamine. This chemical balance may aid in the treatment of anxiety and depression symptoms.

Exercise may cause anatomical changes in the brain, including increased volume in regions related to memory and learning, according to research. As a full-body exercise, Nordic Walking activates numerous muscle groups and increases blood flow to the brain, leading to improved cognitive performance and mental resilience.

Stress Resilience and Coping Strategies: Regular physical exercise, such as Nordic Walking, helps to build stress resilience and effective coping strategies. Individuals get a feeling of success by testing their bodies in a controlled atmosphere, enhancing self-esteem and confidence in their capacity to conquer obstacles in both physical exercise and everyday life.

Outdoor Activities Have Cognitive Benefits:

Cognitive Benefits Of Outdoor Activities

Nordic Walking provides cognitive advantages in addition to stress reduction. Improved attention, creativity, and general cognitive performance have been related to natural surroundings. Physical activity combined with exposure to the outdoors improves mental clarity and attention.

Mind-Body Connection: Nordic Walking stresses the mind-body connection by challenging participants to coordinate their motions with the walking rhythm and pole use. This concerted effort promotes attention and awareness, as well as a sense of flow that is beneficial to mental health.

Nordic Walking as an outdoor sport has the potential to be therapeutic for those coping with a variety of mental health issues. Incorporating this kind of exercise into mental health treatment regimens may supplement standard therapy treatments, providing a more comprehensive approach to well-being.

In conclusion, Nordic Walking treatment shows great potential for improving mental and emotional well-being. This exercise form's blend of physical activity, exposure to the environment, and social factors gives a complete approach to stress reduction, enhanced mental health, and cognitive advantages. As evidence for Nordic Walking's beneficial effect grows, incorporating it into holistic health and wellness practices becomes an increasingly important method for improving overall quality of life.

CHAPTER FIVE

Integrating Nordic Walking Into A Healthy Lifestyle

Integrating Nordic Walking into a healthy lifestyle may provide a varied approach to physical fitness, mental well-being, and general health with the goal of holistic well-being. This chapter delves into the idea of integrating Nordic Walking into everyday routines, creating individualized training schedules, and offering important dietary and hydration advice to maximize the therapeutic advantages of this enjoyable outdoor activity.

Designing Personalized Exercise Plans

1. .Goal Setting and Assessment:

• Evaluate the individual's fitness level, health situation, and particular objectives thoroughly.

• Establish reasonable and attainable goals, taking into account aspects such as weight management, cardiovascular health, and total fitness development.

2. .Nordic Walking Programs Can Be Customized:

• Individualize Nordic Walking programs by including aspects such as length, intensity, and frequency.

• As the individual's fitness increases, gradually raise the complexity of the workout schedule.

3. .Strength and flexibility training should be included:

• To develop a well-rounded training regimen, combining Nordic Walking with strength and flexibility workouts.

• To improve general physical strength and flexibility, include bodyweight exercises, resistance training, and stretching.

4. .Variation and Periodization:

• Use periodization methods to avoid plateaus and improve performance.

• Change up your walking routes, terrains, and intensities to keep your workout interesting and difficult.

5. .Monitoring and modifying:

• Evaluate progress regularly and make any changes to the training regimen.

• Be aware of any physical restrictions or health issues and adjust your approach appropriately.

Nutrition And Hydration Tips

1. .Nutrition Before Walking:

• Before Nordic Walking, eat a balanced meal that includes carbs, proteins, and healthy fats.

• If you're going for a stroll soon after eating, choose easy-to-digest snacks.

2. .Recommendations for Hydration:

• Drink plenty of water before, during, and after Nordic Walking.

• When considering fluid intake, consider weather conditions and individual sweat rates.

3. .After-Walking Recovery:

• Consume a protein- and carbohydrate-rich snack or meal after your walk to aid muscle recovery.

• Replace lost fluids by rehydrating with water or electrolyte-rich drinks.

4. .Supplements for nutrition:

• Determine if you require supplements such as vitamins or minerals, and speak with a healthcare expert if necessary.

• Maintain a well-balanced diet that matches individual nutritional needs.

Incorporating Nordic Walking Into Daily Routines

1. .Transportation and commuting:

• Encourage people to walk to work or include Nordic Walking into their everyday commute habits.

• Think about walking meetings or walking breaks throughout the day.

2. .Social Involvement:

• Organize Nordic Walking groups or clubs to foster a feeling of community.

• Take advantage of social events to go on group walks, encouraging social contact and well-being.

3. .Family and Recreational Activities:

• Incorporate Nordic Walking into family trips or recreational activities.

• Make physical exercise a communal and joyful experience by organizing weekend treks or nature excursions.

4. .Mindful Walking Techniques:

•   Highlight   Nordic   Walking's contemplative   features,   encouraging participants to be present in the moment.

• Incorporate mindfulness practices, such as focused breathing, into your walking sessions to improve your mental health.

5. .Environmental Concerns:

•   Encourage   ecologically   beneficial activities   by   opting   for   green transportation   or   arranging environmentally aware walking events.

• During Nordic Walking programs, encourage participants to enjoy and connect with nature.

To summarize, incorporating Nordic Walking into a healthy lifestyle requires careful planning, tailored methods of exercise, a mindful diet, and innovative integration into everyday routines. Individuals may utilize the therapeutic advantages of Nordic Walking by adhering to these guidelines to attain overall well-being and an enhanced quality of life.

CHAPTER SIX

Nordic Walking For Special Populations

Nordic Walking is a flexible physical exercise that may be tailored to meet the specific demands of different groups. This chapter delves into the many adaptations and advantages of Nordic Walking for elders, those undergoing rehabilitation, and people suffering from chronic diseases.

Adaptations For Seniors

1. . Modifications to the Equipment:
Seniors may readily adapt to Nordic Walking by using lighter poles and changing the length to guarantee good

posture and stability. To address any grip constraints, ergonomic handles with pleasant grips may be added.

2. . Pace and Intensity:

Seniors may need to work at a lesser intensity and a slower pace. Individualizing the intensity of exercise to an individual's fitness level and gradually increasing it over time helps to reduce strain and improves commitment to the activity.

3. . Exercises for Balance and Stability:

Seniors might benefit from including particular balance and stability exercises in their Nordic Walking regimens.

This improves proprioception and lowers the chance of falling, which is especially essential in this age range.

4. . Aspects of Society:

Nordic Walking may also be used as a social activity for the elderly. Group sessions build a sense of community, minimizing feelings of isolation and giving emotional support, all of which contribute to members' overall well-being.

Nordic Walking And Rehabilitation

1. . Low-Intensity Exercise:

Nordic Walking is a low-impact exercise option for those in rehabilitation. The method spreads the stress throughout the whole body, limiting joint impact and the danger of worsening problems.

2. . Muscle Activity and Rehabilitation:

Nordic Walking's distinctive movement pattern utilizes a broad variety of muscles, making it a useful tool for rehabilitation. This participation may help to regain strength, flexibility, and coordination, enabling a more complete recovery.

3. . Therapeutic Advantages:

Nordic walking has been acknowledged for its therapeutic advantages, which include better cardiovascular health and pulmonary function. These advantages may be quite beneficial in the rehabilitation process, particularly for those recuperating from cardiovascular or respiratory disorders.

4. . Implementation in Physical Therapy Programs:

Nordic Walking is easily incorporated into physical treatment regimens. Physical therapists may utilize this exercise to supplement other therapy methods, allowing them to provide a more comprehensive approach to recovery.

Benefits For Individuals With Chronic Conditions

1. . Cardiovascular Wellness:
Nordic walking has been demonstrated to improve heart and lung function, hence improving cardiovascular health.

Individuals with chronic diseases such as heart disease or diabetes might benefit from adopting Nordic Walking into their regimen to improve their overall cardiovascular well-being.

2. . Health of the Joints:

Nordic Walking's low-impact nature is especially beneficial for those who have chronic joint ailments like arthritis. The uniform distribution of pressure on the joints reduces stress and allows for joint-friendly activity.

3. . Psychological Health:
Nordic Walking may have a favorable impact on one's mental health. The rhythmic activity, exposure to the outdoors, and social features of group

activities help to relieve stress, anxiety, and depression, all of which are typical issues for people with chronic diseases.

4. . Mobility and functional improvement:

Nordic Walking improves general mobility and functioning, making it a good alternative for those who have chronic diseases that limit their ability to move. This activity's full-body involvement may result in enhanced balance, coordination, and flexibility.

Finally, Nordic Walking provides a customized and inclusive approach to physical exercise, making it a powerful tool for increasing health and well-being in a variety of groups, including the elderly, those undergoing rehabilitation, and people with chronic diseases. As academics and practitioners continue to investigate the possible applications of Nordic Walking, its significance in improving the health and quality of life of particular groups becomes clearer.

CHAPTER SEVEN

Exploring Nordic Walking Environments

Nordic Walking Therapy is a comprehensive method that combines the physical advantages of Nordic walking with nature's and social interaction's therapeutic features.

In Chapter Seven, we look into the many settings in which Nordic Walking Therapy is practiced, studying the distinct characteristics of Urban Nordic Walking, Nature Trails and Wilderness Exploration, and the Social characteristics of Group Nordic Walking.

Urban Nordic Walking

By adding the busy downtown into the walking experience, Urban Nordic Walking adds a dynamic layer to the treatment. This atmosphere presents players with a unique mix of difficulties and possibilities. Individuals in metropolitan areas may include Nordic walking into their everyday routines, converting dull treks into meaningful and energizing workout sessions.

The Advantages of Urban Nordic Walking:

1. .**Accessibility:** Urban environments, such as parks, walkways, and promenades, offer accessible venues for Nordic

walking. This makes it simple for people to integrate the exercise into their regular life.

2.   .**Stress Reduction:** Despite the hustle and bustle of city life, Urban Nordic Walking may be a stress-relieving sport. Walking's rhythmic action, along with urban green areas, may add to mental well-being.

3.   .**Community Engagement:** Because urban Nordic walking draws a lot of attention, it opens up chances for community involvement. This may help people feel more connected and supported.

4. **Terrain Variation:** Urban surroundings provide a variety of terrains, ranging from level sidewalks to inclines and stairs.

This variation improves the entire exercise by engaging various muscle groups.

Nature Trails And Wilderness Exploration

Nordic Walking uses nature as a therapeutic background, delivering an immersive experience that promotes both physical and emotional well-being. Nature paths and wilderness regions provide a tranquil and revitalizing setting that compliments the rhythmic activity of Nordic walking.

Nature Trails & Wilderness Exploration Highlights:

1. **.Natural Terrain Obstacles:** Uneven routes, diverse surfaces, and natural obstacles

make for an interesting and hard exercise. This activates stabilizing muscles and improves Nordic walking's overall efficacy.

2. .**Mind-Body Connection:** Spending time in nature helps to strengthen the connection between the mind and the body. During nature-based Nordic Walking Therapy, participants often report increased emotions of awareness and calm.

3. .**Therapeutic Landscapes:** Visual and aural stimulation in natural surroundings add to the activity's therapeutic benefits. This includes nature's soothing noises, the visual splendor of landscapes, and the fresh air.

4.   .**Benefits of Biodiversity:** Exposure to different flora and fauna fosters a feeling of connectedness with the natural world, which contributes to mental well-being. Nordic Walking Therapy may also be used as Eco therapy to promote environmental consciousness.

Social Aspects Of Group Nordic Walking

Nordic Walking Therapy relies heavily on social interaction. Group Nordic walking sessions promote a feeling of community, support, and drive, enhancing the activity's therapeutic advantages.

Social Benefits and Group Dynamics:

1.   **.Motivation and Accountability:** Group sessions create a supportive atmosphere in which participants inspire one another, hence increasing therapeutic adherence. Accountability to the group might promote consistent engagement.

2.   .Group Nordic walking fosters social connection, which reduces feelings of isolation and loneliness. Participants often connect with others who share their interests, forming a supportive group.

3. **.Structured Programs:** Structured programs, such as warm-up exercises, Nordic walking drills, and cool-down routines, may be used to arrange group sessions.

This format increases the therapeutic effect and assures a well-rounded session.

4. .Group Nordic walking has an inviting atmosphere and is appropriate for people of all fitness levels. This openness fosters a feeling of belonging and motivates people to push themselves at their own pace.

Finally, Chapter Seven examines the many venues in which Nordic Walking Therapy takes place, emphasizing the distinct advantages of Urban Nordic Walking, the therapeutic aspects of Nature Trails and Wilderness Exploration, and the significance of the Social Aspects within group settings.

CHAPTER EIGHT

Nordic Walking Events And Communities

Nordic Walking, which has its origins in cross-country skiing, has grown in popularity as a low-impact, full-body workout ideal for people of all ages and fitness levels. Nordic Walking has generated a thriving community of aficionados who gather together via events, clubs, and organizations, in addition to its health advantages. This chapter discusses the relevance of Nordic Walking events and the feeling of community they foster, the advantages of joining clubs and organizations, and the value of developing a supporting network.

Participating In Nordic Walking Events

1. . Event Variety and Inclusion:

Nordic Walking events range from strolls to competitive races, making the sport accessible to individuals of all fitness levels and aspirations. Because activities often cater to novices, seasoned walkers, and individuals with special health concerns, inclusivity is an important aspect.

2. . Community Development:

Participating in Nordic Walking events allows folks to meet other Nordic Walking aficionados.

Because participants have a shared passion for health, fitness, and the outdoors, these activities generate a feeling of belonging.

3. . Expos for Health and Wellness:

Many Nordic Walking events have health and wellness expos where attendees may learn about the most recent equipment, methods, and breakthroughs in the industry. These expos help to educate the community by advocating a holistic approach to well-being.

4. . Interaction with Others:
Nordic Walking activities are more than just a form of fitness; they are also social gatherings. Participants often form new acquaintances, share advice and

experiences, and form long-lasting ties, reinforcing the feeling of community.

5. . Charity and Fundraising Activities:

Some Nordic Walking events are planned as charity walks or fundraisers, allowing participants to donate to worthwhile organizations while exercising. This gives the community a charitable component.

Joining Nordic Walking Clubs And Groups

1. . Training Programs with Structure:

Nordic Walking clubs often provide organized training programs for people of various ability levels. Joining a club gives you access to professional advice, which may help you improve your technique, posture, and general health.

2. . Shared Knowledge and Experiences:

Being a member of a club allows you to share your experiences and learn from other walkers. Members may share advice, discuss obstacles, and celebrate accomplishments, fostering a positive learning atmosphere.

3. . Planned Group Walks:

Club-organized group walks provide a systematic and structured approach to Nordic Walking. These walks create a social atmosphere in which participants may enjoy the outdoors while benefitting from the incentive that group activities give.

4. . Sense of Responsibility:

Joining a Nordic Walking group instills a feeling of responsibility. Knowing that others are looking forward to your involvement in a group walk may be a tremendous incentive, assuring regular engagement and improvement.

Building A Supportive Community

1. . Social Media and Online Platforms:

Building a supportive community entails more than just physical meetings. Nordic Walking groups often flourish on internet platforms and social media, where members may exchange information, seek assistance, and motivate one another on their fitness journeys.

2. . Programs for Mentoring:

Mentorship programs established within Nordic Walking groups enable experienced walkers to assist newbies. This creates a welcoming atmosphere in which information and encouragement are shared, supporting development and inclusion.

3. . Community Activities Other Than Walking:

Nordic Walking groups may enhance friendships by organizing activities other than walking, such as picnics, seminars, or health retreats. These activities provide a comprehensive feeling of well-being and help to enhance the community's social fabric.

4. . Celebrations and Recognition:

Recognizing individual accomplishments and celebrating communal milestones fosters a pleasant environment. Recognizing achievement, whether it's a personal fitness goal or a community-wide accomplishment, develops a feeling of pride and solidarity.

Finally, Nordic Walking events and communities play an important role in improving practitioners' overall experience.

The inclusive character of events, the educational opportunities they provide, the advantages of joining clubs, and the feeling of community established around shared interests all contribute considerably to the overall well-being of Nordic Walkers. As the community grows, the connections formed via events and groups become essential components of a supporting network that promotes a healthy and active lifestyle.

CHAPTER NINE

Scientific Research And Nordic Walking

Nordic Walking Therapy has gained popularity in recent years as a possible treatment for a variety of physical and mental health concerns. This chapter examines the scientific research on Nordic Walking Therapy, offering an overview of study results, summarizing current investigations, and recommending future research paths. Expert advice and suggestions from healthcare experts and researchers in the area will also be considered.

Numerous research studies have been conducted to investigate the impact of Nordic Walking Therapy on various demographics and health issues. The following are the major study results summarized:

1. .Cardiovascular Advantages:

• Scientific evidence repeatedly shows that Nordic Walking improves cardiovascular health. When opposed to regular walking, the use of poles stimulates upper body muscles, boosting heart rate and oxygen consumption.

• Research has shown that it improves blood pressure, cholesterol levels, and general cardiovascular fitness.

2. .Musculoskeletal Wellness:

• Nordic Walking has been linked to improved musculoskeletal health. The use of poles more uniformly distributes the burden across the body, decreasing stress on joints and muscles.

• Studies show that Nordic Walking improves posture, balance, and strength, making it a helpful treatment for those suffering from illnesses like osteoarthritis.

3. .Mental Health Advantages:

• Evidence demonstrates that Nordic Walking Therapy improves mental well-being. The combination of physical exercise and outdoor exposure helps to alleviate stress, anxiety, and depression symptoms.

• Research has looked at its potential as a supplementary therapy for mental health issues, especially when combined with standard therapies.

4. .Chronic Illnesses:

• Nordic Walking has been investigated as an adjuvant treatment for a variety of chronic illnesses such as diabetes, obesity, and chronic obstructive pulmonary disease (COPD).

• Studies show benefits in metabolic indicators, weight control, and respiratory function.

While current research is useful, further study is needed to have a better knowledge of Nordic Walking Therapy. Current and future research priorities include:

1. .**Populations of Interest:**

• Researching the effectiveness of Nordic Walking in certain demographics, such as older persons, those with neurological problems, or those in rehabilitation, may give unique insights for these groups.

2. .Long-Term Consequences:

• Longitudinal studies are required to establish the long-term advantages of Nordic Walking. Understanding the long-term effects on cardiovascular health, musculoskeletal function, and mental well-being is critical for encouraging its usage.

3. .Comparative Research:

• Comparative studies comparing Nordic Walking to other kinds of exercise or therapeutic therapies may aid in determining its relative efficacy and acceptability for various persons and circumstances.

4. .Action Mechanisms:

• Research into the physiological and psychological factors underpinning Nordic Walking may help us better understand how it delivers therapeutic benefits. This information may be used to guide focused treatments and enhance treatment results.

Expert Opinions And Recommendations

Experts in the area share their knowledge and ideas for incorporating Nordic Walking Therapy into clinical practice:

1. .Taking a Multidisciplinary Approach:

• Experts underline the necessity of using a multidisciplinary approach to personalize Nordic Walking programs to individual requirements, engaging physiotherapists, exercise physiologists, and mental health experts.

2. .Training and education:

• Nordic Walking instructors and healthcare professionals should attend training programs to ensure proper technique and program design. This guarantees that Nordic Walking Therapy is implemented safely and effectively.

3. .Public Education:

• Experts emphasize the need to raise public knowledge about the advantages of Nordic Walking, promoting it as an accessible and fun form of exercise suited for people of all ages and fitness levels.

4. .Advocacy for Public Policy:

• It is advised to advocate for the incorporation of Nordic Walking Therapy into public health policies and initiatives. This includes promoting its incorporation in community-based wellness and rehabilitation efforts.

Finally, Nordic Walking Therapy seems to be a promising comprehensive strategy for improving physical and mental well-being. Ongoing research will further prove its effectiveness, refine its use across varied groups, and contribute to its inclusion into mainstream healthcare practices, driven by expert views and suggestions.

CHAPTER TEN

The Future Of Nordic Walking Therapy

Nordic Walking Therapy has grown in popularity as a comprehensive approach to physical and mental health. As we look to the future of this therapeutic activity, it is critical to investigate new trends, possible uses in healthcare, and advocacy methods to promote Nordic Walking on a worldwide scale.

Emerging Trends And Innovations

1. .**Integration of Smart Devices and Wearables:** As technology advances, the incorporation of smart devices and wearables into Nordic Walking may

improve the entire experience. Sensor-enabled poles, smart clothes, and smartphone apps may offer real-time input on posture, stride, and intensity, enabling people and therapists to measure progress and tailor therapies.

2. .Immersive technology such as virtual reality (VR) and augmented reality (AR) may be used in Nordic Walking Therapy to create engaging and therapeutic experiences. Virtual landscapes may imitate varied terrains, improving the whole experience and making treatment more fun for people of varying fitness levels and tastes.

3. .Biofeedback devices may assess physiological responses such as heart rate,

muscular tension, and breathing patterns. By incorporating these technologies into Nordic Walking, users may get rapid feedback, increasing self-awareness and enhancing the therapeutic advantages of each session.

4.   **.Personalized Nordic Walking Training Programs:** Advanced data analytics and artificial intelligence may be used to create customized Nordic Walking training programs. These programs may take into account individual health profiles, preferences, and progress over time, ensuring that treatment is personalized to each participant's specific requirements.

1.   .Nordic Walking Therapy has the potential to become an essential component of rehabilitation programs, assisting in the recovery of those suffering from injuries or procedures. Because of its low-impact nature and ability to stimulate numerous muscle groups, it is an excellent choice for rehabilitation and injury prevention.

2.   **.Chronic Disease Management:** Nordic Walking's therapeutic effects may be used to manage chronic disorders such as cardiovascular disease, diabetes, and arthritis. According to research, frequent Nordic Walking may enhance

cardiovascular fitness, blood glucose levels, and joint mobility, making it an important component of comprehensive healthcare programs.

3.   .**Mental Health and Well-Being:** Nordic Walking has been shown to improve mental health by lowering stress, anxiety, and depression. In the future, Nordic Walking Therapy might be included in mental health treatment regimens, wellness programs, and stress management efforts.

Advocacy And Promoting Nordic Walking On A Global Scale

1.   .**Professional Training and Certification:** Creating standardized training programs and certifications for Nordic Walking teachers and therapists may help the treatment gain legitimacy and popularity. Collaboration with health organizations, fitness institutions, and rehabilitation clinics is required to guarantee that Nordic Walking programs are led by trained specialists.

2.   .**Research & Evidence-Based Practice:** It is critical to do ongoing research into the therapeutic effects of Nordic Walking and its applicability in diverse healthcare settings.

Building a strong body of evidence will make it easier to incorporate Nordic Walking into mainstream healthcare practices, gaining support from medical experts and legislators.

3. .**Campaigns for Public Awareness:** Advocacy activities should include public awareness campaigns to educate people about the advantages of Nordic Walking Therapy. Collaboration with healthcare experts, fitness enthusiasts, and community groups may aid in the promotion of the practice as a viable and accessible therapeutic choice.

4.   .**worldwide Events and Collaborations:** Organizing worldwide Nordic Walking events, conferences, and collaborations

may help practitioners and enthusiasts build a feeling of community. This may also be used to communicate research results, exchange ideas, and highlight success stories, all of which contribute to the worldwide promotion of Nordic Walking Therapy.

To summarize, the future of Nordic Walking Therapy seems bright, with rising trends, creative uses in healthcare, and advocacy initiatives all playing important roles in the therapy's continuous expansion and acceptance as a holistic therapeutic approach. Nordic Walking has the potential to become a widespread intervention for physical and mental well-being on a worldwide scale as technology and research advance.

Conclusion

Nordic walking therapy has developed as a viable strategy that combines physical exercise with the serenity of nature to promote overall well-being. In conclusion, this novel therapy has numerous advantages that go beyond standard therapies.

Walking with specially constructed poles not only improves cardiovascular fitness but also works a broader variety of muscles, making it an enticing alternative for anyone looking for low-impact yet effective training. Furthermore, rhythmic exercise, when combined with being outside, has mental health benefits, lowering stress, anxiety, and depression while fostering a feeling of peace and connection with nature.

Nordic walking therapy's accessibility and versatility make it a flexible alternative for a wide range of demographics, including those recovering from injuries, managing chronic ailments, or just looking to enhance their general health. Its social component enhances the experience by promoting group engagement and cultivating a supportive community.

Nordic walking therapy is a testimony to the synergy between physical exercise, nature, and mental well-being, as research continues to reveal its advantages. Its incorporation into therapeutic methods might serve as a complementary approach to traditional therapies, providing a holistic approach to health improvement.

However, further research is needed to investigate its usefulness across diverse groups and health situations. Understanding its long-term influence and improving implementation guidelines may assist in optimizing its therapeutic potential.

Finally, Nordic walking therapy has the potential as an integrated strategy to improve overall well-being by exploiting the natural advantages of physical activity and environmental immersion. Its rise emphasizes the significance of investigating innovative ways that promote not just physical health, but also mental and emotional well-being, opening the way for a more complete approach to healthcare.

THE END

www.ingramcontent.com/pod-product-compliance
Lightning Source LLC
Chambersburg PA
CBHW050737260726
48661CB00001B/285